Ovarian Cyst

All You Need To Know

Dr. Sheila Harrison

Disclaimer

This content serves to provide general information about the disease and aims to empower you to seek prompt medical assistance if necessary to prevent complications. It's essential to stress that this information is not a substitute for consulting a qualified physician. The field of medical science is continually evolving, and due to the dynamic nature of medical knowledge, we recommend seeking expert advice if you encounter any inconsistencies or intend to take action based on the information in this content. Never disregard professional medical guidance or delay treatment based on something you've read online, including this material, or from any other online source. Always remember that the internet cannot cure you; rather, healing comes through the guidance of medical professionals and the providence of God.

NOTICE: *Reader Descretion is Advised due to nature of some of the image Content Of the book. Thank You.*

Table of Content

Section 1

Overview

An ovarian cyst is a fluid-filled sac that grows in the ovary during ovulation. They usually occur within or on the surface of the ovaries, part of the female reproductive system which produces hormones oestrogen and progesterone, as well as egg cells (ova) needed for reproduction. Ovarian cysts are common and affect women of all ages, even after menopause. Most ovarian cysts that form are benign and will shrink on their own after some time.

Benign cysts do not cause any pain or discomfort, but some cysts may be at risk of rupturing. Ruptured cysts can lead to a host of complications that require immediate medical attention. An ovarian cyst could also be a risk factor for ovarian cancer.

Most of these cysts disappear during the first 14 to 16 weeks of pregnancy, but some, such as theca lutein cysts, can persist until delivery. The majority of these cystic masses are non-functional after 16 weeks of pregnancy.

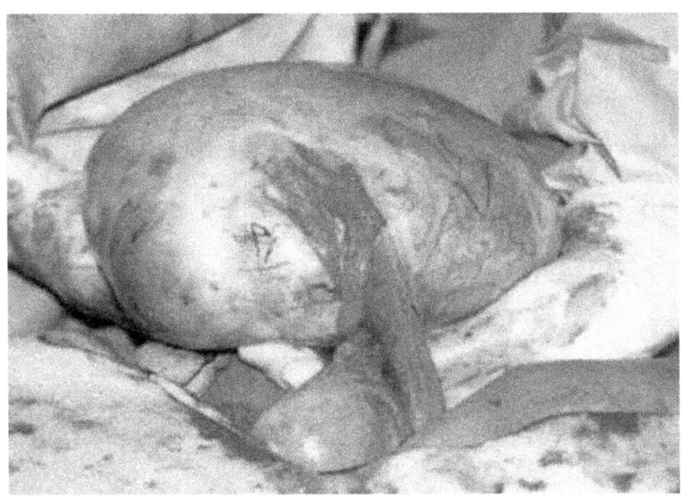

Image above is a multilocular right ovarian cyst that is 24 cm in lemgth

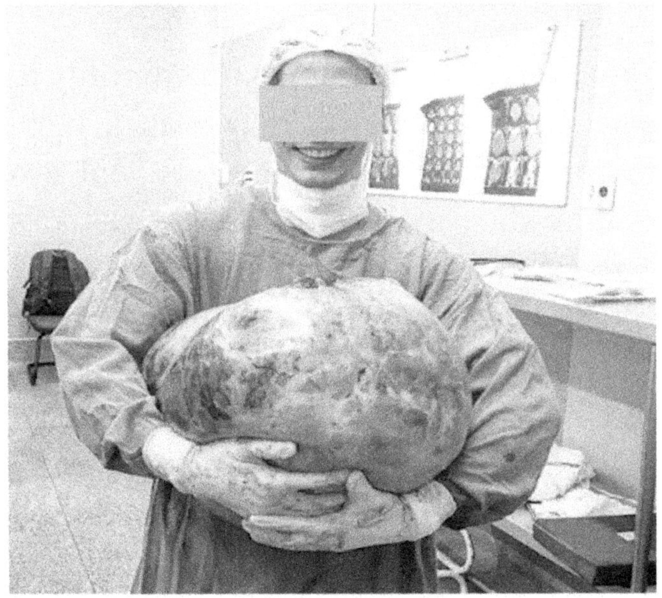

Section 2

Types and Causes of Ovarian Cysts

Functional cysts and **pathological cysts** are the two main types of ovarian cysts. The two most common types of functional ovarian cysts are corpus luteum and follicular cysts. Cysts associated with endometriosis, dermoid cysts, and cystadenoma cysts make up the majority of the pathological cysts.

Functional cysts, the most commonly diagnosed type of ovarian cyst, occur as a result of the normal function of the menstrual cycle. They usually start from a follicle, a cyst-like structure that produces egg cells. Normally, a mature follicle, or sac, breaks open to release an egg. After the egg is released, the follicle dissolves and becomes a corpus luteum, which produces oestrogen and progesterone. An ovarian cyst forms when the follicle, or corpus luteum, has a defect that causes it to accumulate liquid and thus form a cyst.

There are two types of functional cysts.

- **Follicle cysts:** This form when the follicle does not break open to release an egg and causes a build-up of liquid, forming a cyst.
- **Corpus luteum cysts**: This occur after the follicle has become a corpus luteum, but a build-up of liquid causes it to form a cyst.

The most common ovarian masses associated with pregnancy are functional cysts, such as the corpus luteum of pregnancy and theca-lutein cysts. On ultrasound, hormonal factors can cause the follicular cyst or corpus luteum cyst to appear differently.

Functional cysts are the most common, but are usually harmless and cause no symptoms. These will often shrink and disappear after two or three menstrual cycles. Functional cysts also do not occur in menopausal women since their ovaries no longer produce eggs.

There are also other types of uncommon ovarian cysts that are not related to the menstrual cycle. These cysts mainly form due to abnormal cell growth.

- **Dermoid cysts**: These cysts contain tissue (hair, skin, fatty tissue, etc.), as they are formed from embryonic cells. They are also known as teratomas. These benign cysts generally grow to rather large sizes, and must be surgically removed.

- **Cystadenomas**: These are formed from cells lining the exterior of the ovaries, growing outside while attached to the ovaries by a stalk-like structure. They may contain a watery or mucous-like material, and can also grow to a rather large size.

- **Endometriomas**: These cysts are caused by endometriosis, a medical condition where uterine endometrial tissue – tissue similar to the lining of the uterus – grows outside of the womb. These are referred to as "chocolate cysts" due to the colour of blood found within the cysts.

Both dermoid cysts and cystadenomas may be harmless, but exceptionally large ones can move the ovary out of position and cause ovarian torsion. This is when an ovary twists around the ligaments holding it in place. Ovarian torsion is very dangerous, as it cuts off blood supply to the ovary and the fallopian tube (the structure that carries ova from the ovary to the uterus).

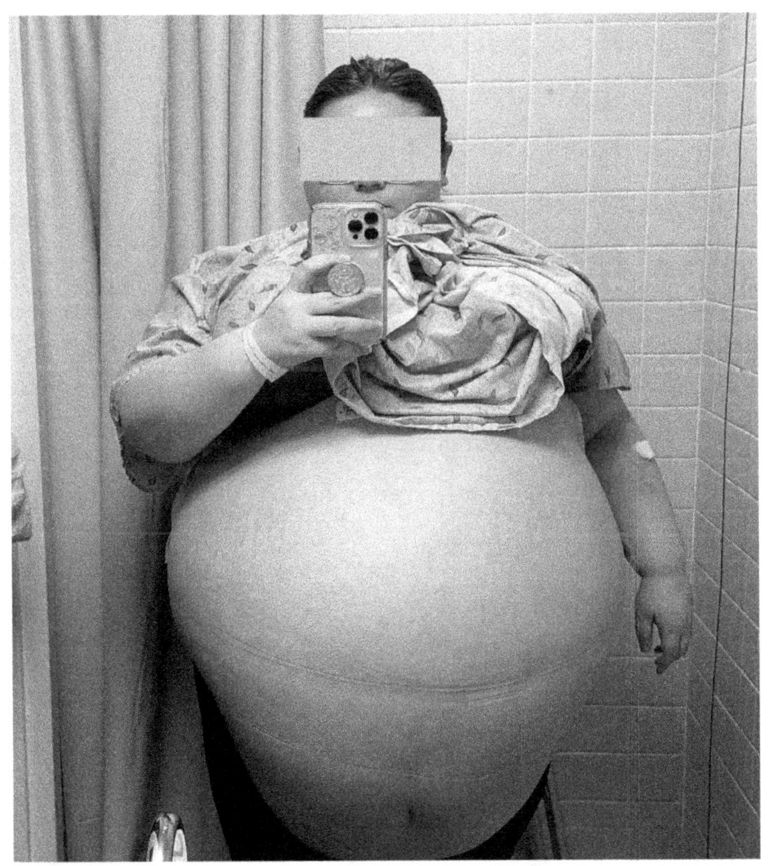

Section 3

Risk Factors of Ovarian Cysts

A person can be at risk of having an ovarian cyst if they have any of the following risk factors:

- Hormonal imbalance, or other hormonal issues
- Pregnancy (a cyst that persists on the ovary even after ovulation)
- Having endometriosis (where uterine endometrial cells grow outside the uterus)
- Having polycystic ovary syndrome (PCOS)
- Severe pelvic infection
- Smoking
- Hypothyroidism (low thyroid hormones in the body)
- A previous ovarian cyst
- Bleeding

Note that having any of these risk factors does not mean that you will develop an ovarian cyst.

Bleeding in ovarian cyst

There are various types of ovarian cysts. Most of them are usually discovered incidentally on physical examination or imaging. Ovarian cysts can cause complications, including rupture, hemorrhage, and torsion, which are considered gynecological emergencies.

Yes, it is possible. Depending on the type of cyst and its size, bleeding can occur due to different reasons. It's important to note that not all ovarian cysts cause bleeding, and many of them may not result in any symptom at all. However, if you experience sudden or severe pelvic pain, heavy bleeding, or other unusual symptoms, it's important to seek medical attention right away.

There are various ways through which it can result in bleeding.

- One of the most common reasons is that a cyst can interfere with the normal function of the ovaries, leading to hormonal imbalances. Specifically, ovarian cysts can produce hormones such as estrogen or progesterone, which can affect the menstrual cycle. Thus, leading to problems with the menstrual cycle, such as heavy or irregular periods, or spotting (abnormal vaginal bleeding between periods). If a cyst produces excessive estrogen, it can cause the lining of the uterus to thicken, leading to heavier or prolonged periods. On the other hand, if a cyst interferes with the production of progesterone, it can cause irregular or missed periods.

- In some cases, an ovarian cyst can rupture or twist, leading to sudden and severe pain and bleeding. A ruptured ovarian cyst can also cause bleeding. When it bursts open, it can cause severe pain and bleeding inside the pelvis. This needs immediate medical attention. This can also lead to complications such as internal bleeding or infection.
- Additionally, bleeding can also occur if a type of ovarian cyst, known as hemorrhagic cysts, are filled with blood ruptures.

Section 4

Symptoms of Ovarian Cysts

Most patients with ovarian cysts are asymptomatic, with the cysts being discovered incidentally during ultrasonography or routine pelvic examination. Some cysts, however, may be associated with a range of symptoms, sometimes severe, including the following [1]:

- Pain or discomfort in the lower abdomen

- Abdominal swelling

- Severe pain from torsion (twisting) or rupture - Cyst rupture is characterized by sudden, sharp, unilateral pelvic pain; this can be associated with trauma, exercise, or coitus. Cyst rupture can lead to peritoneal signs, abdominal distention, and bleeding (which is usually self-limited)

- Discomfort with intercourse, particularly deep penetration

- Changes in bowel movements such as constipation

- Pelvic pressure causing tenesmus or urinary frequency

- Menstrual irregularities

- Nausea or vomiting

- Difficulty urinating, or a frequent need to urinate

- Fullness even after eating small portions

- Difficulty in getting pregnant

- Precocious puberty and early menarche in young children

- Abdominal fullness and bloating

- Indigestion, heartburn, or early satiety

- Endometriomas: These are associated with endometriosis, which causes a classic triad of painful and heavy periods and dyspareunia

- Tachycardia and hypotension: These may result from hemorrhage caused by cyst rupture

- Hyperpyrexia: This may result from some complications of ovarian cysts, such as ovarian torsion [1]

- Adnexal or cervical motion tenderness

- Underlying malignancy may be associated with early satiety, weight loss/cachexia, lymphadenopathy, or shortness of breath related to ascites or pleural effusion

Benign ovarian cysts do not cause any adverse symptoms until they rupture, are of a large size, and/or block blood supply to the ovaries. If any of the above occurs, symptoms that can present themselves may include (but are not limited to):

If you or your loved one suffers sudden, severe pain, it could be a sign that the cyst has either ruptured or ovarian torsion has occurred. A ruptured cyst can lead to internal bleeding, which will require immediate medical attention.

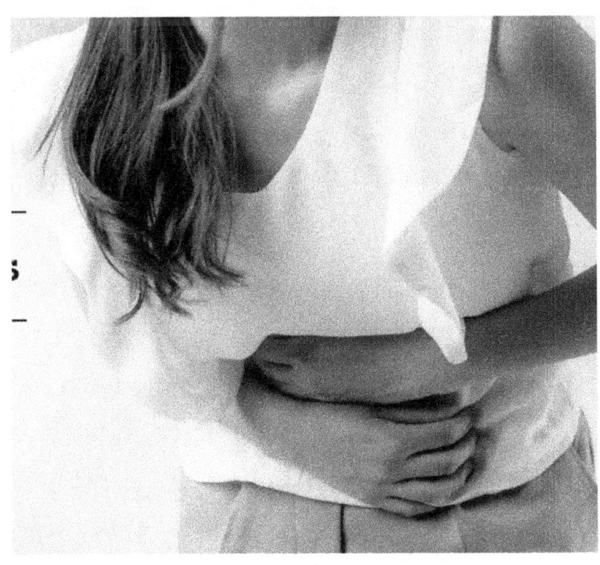

Section 5

Diagnosing Ovarian Cysts

As most ovarian cysts are harmless, they often go undiagnosed and eventually disappear after some time. In some instances, women being examined for other medical reasons may incidentally discover the presence of an asymptomatic ovarian cyst. If you or your loved one are having any of its symptoms, though, this may indicate the presence of a large or malignant cyst.

A routine pelvic examination by a doctor is the first step to making a diagnosis. For this examination, the doctor will examine you or your loved one's reproductive organs and make sure that nothing is out of the ordinary. They will usually try to detect any abnormal lumps or changes that they can feel.

Your doctor may order a pelvic ultrasound for further examination. This is much like a pregnancy ultrasound test, but for checking you or your loved one's reproductive system. The ultrasound scan will be performed to confirm if there really is a cyst, where it is located, how large its size is and whether it is solid, filled with fluid, or a mix of both.

Other diagnosis methods may include:

- **Laparoscopy**: The doctor makes a small incision on the abdomen and inserts a slim instrument with a small light and camera (a laparoscope) to examine the ovaries. As this is a surgical method, you or your loved one will be under anaesthesia. If a cyst is detected, the doctor may also remove it during this procedure.

- **CT/MRI scan**: If the ultrasound is unable to yield results, a CT or MRI scan may be done instead. An MRI scan uses magnetic waves to produce detailed images of your internal organs, while a CT scan uses body imaging to create a cross-section of your internal organs.

- **CA125 blood test**: This test looks for a specific protein called cancer antigen 125, or CA125, in your bloodstream. The presence of this protein in your blood can be an early marker for ovarian cancer but is not necessarily accurate. Further tests may need to be done to confirm if it is cancer or otherwise.

Section 6

Ovarian Cysts in Pregnancy

The corpus luteum is responsible for progesterone production during pregnancy and normally regresses at around 8 weeks' gestation.

Most pregnancy-associated cysts, such as corpus luteal and follicular cysts, resolve by gestational age 14-16 weeks and are hormonally responsive, allowing conservative management. By gestational age 16-20 weeks, up to 96% of masses resolve spontaneously. Resolution of cysts are less likely when larger than 5cm or of complex morphology. Simple cysts smaller than 6 cm in diameter have a risk of malignancy of less than 1%.

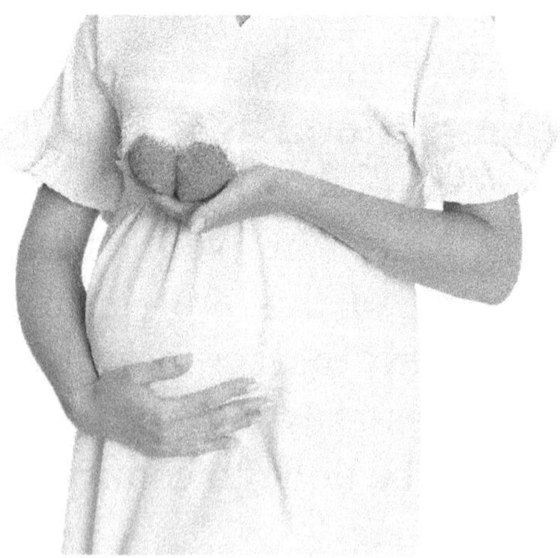

Corpus luteal cysts tend to be larger and more symptomatic than follicular cysts and are more prone to hemorrhage and rupture. Follicular cysts are usually smaller, with internal hemorrhage being relatively uncommon.

Masses that persist longer may warrant further workup for potential neoplastic disease based on clinical findings and radiologic evidence. Serum CA125 studies are not recommended in pregnancy, as levels can fluctuate widely in normal pregnancy, particularly in the first and second trimesters, and can be elevated in many benign conditions. One group suggests observation, with postpartum surgery in select patients who have large, persistent adnexal masses in whom ultrasonographic findings are not highly suggestive of malignancy. However, in situations in which cysts are symptomatic, including causing pain and discomfort, or with rapid growth on serial ultrasound, surgical removal should be considered.

If malignancy is a possibility and peripartum surgery is warranted, the risk of harming the pregnancy is weighed against a delay in treatment, but surgery is generally delayed until the mid-second trimester, when most cysts have resolved.

Some ovarian conditions unique to pregnancy include the hyperstimulated ovary, ovarian hyperstimulation syndrome, hyperreactio luteinalis, theca-lutein cysts, and luteoma of pregnancy. Hyperstimulated ovaries represent a normal ovarian response to circulating hCG levels and are typically seen in women who have undergone ovulation induction.

Pregnancy-related ovarian cyst bursts

Even when pregnant, a functional ovarian cyst rupture is typically not a cause for concern. With time, the cyst's fluid will naturally reabsorb, so all that is required is some pain relief medication and a few days of pelvic rest.
In fact, the majority of medical professionals advise against treating ruptured ovarian cysts during pregnancy other than with watchful waiting, which entails observation, ultrasounds, and monitoring.

Although not all women experience pain following an ovarian cyst rupture, some do. An ovarian cyst rupture can cause moderate to severe pain, vaginal bleeding, nausea, vomiting, lightheadedness, and even fever.

However, if there is a risk of infection from the rupture, significant bleeding, torsion, or another effect on the pregnancy in some way, your doctor may advise surgery.

What can a pregnant woman do if she has an ovarian cyst?

The majority of ovarian cysts won't affect your pregnancy in any way. For instance, the chances are good that a corpus luteum cyst will disappear on its own by the second trimester. While some other types of cysts may continue to grow during pregnancy and occasionally cause pain, most of the time these cysts don't harm the fetus.

In order to ensure that an ovarian cyst won't affect your pregnancy, ask your doctor to schedule routine ultrasounds to check your ovaries. An ovarian cyst ultrasound can be used to keep track of any cyst to make sure it doesn't develop or change in a way that might be alarming.

Fetal and Neonatal Cysts

In female newborns, ovarian cysts are the most frequent type of abdominal tumor, with an estimated incidence of more than 30%.

Fetal ovarian cysts are believed to be caused by hormonal stimulation, such as fetal gonadotropins, maternal estrogen, and placental hCG. In addition, an association between fetal ovarian cysts and maternal diabetes and fetal hypothyroidism has been identified.

Most fetal ovarian cysts are small and involute within the first few months of life and are not of clinical significance. They are generally diagnosed in the third trimester of pregnancy, and most tend to resolve at 2-10 weeks postnatally.

Differential diagnoses of these cysts include urachal cysts, intestinal duplication abnormalities, cystic teratoma, and intestinal obstruction. Intrauterine ultrasonography is necessary to differentiate ovarian cysts from these other possibilities.

Aspiration of these cysts can be performed but is associated with complications, such as reformation of cyst, infection, and premature labor. Once the diagnosis of a fetal ovarian cyst is made, it is important to perform serial ultrasonographic examinations to detect any structural changes in size or appearance or complications, such as hydramnios, ascites, or torsion. Of these complications, ovarian torsion is the most serious complication of a fetal ovarian cyst and may manifest as fetal tachycardia due to peritoneal irritation.

Proper management includes serial ultrasonography to look for signs of regression or postnatal surgery if the cyst is complicated or larger than 5 cm in diameter.

Ovarian Cysts in Postmenopausal Women

While functional cysts rarely occur in postmenopausal women, they are still at risk from other types of ovarian cysts. Even though the ovaries are no longer actively producing eggs or hormones, they are still active and thus, at risk of developing cysts. A study estimates that by age 65, approximately 4% of women will be hospitalised for ovarian cysts.

The symptoms and risk factors of ovarian cysts in postmenopausal women are similar to those that occur in premenopausal women. However, the risk of ovarian cancer is high in postmenopausal women. As such, the doctor may order a specific test to look out for cancer markers (refer to the Diagnosing Ovarian Cysts below) in order to determine if the cyst is malignant or otherwise. An ultrasound imaging test may also be performed. Treating the cyst may differ depending on the nature of the cyst.

Ovarian Cysts VS Polycystic Ovary Syndrome (PCOS)

Having prolonged symptoms listed above could be a sign of polycystic ovary syndrome, or PCOS. PCOS is a medical disorder where the ovaries' functions are impaired and cause hormonal imbalance. The three main features of PCOS are:

1. Irregular and/or prolonged periods (or none at all) which disrupt the ovulation process;

2. Abnormal levels of male sex hormones (androgens) which cause physical changes such as excess facial or body hair;

3. Polycystic ovaries, where the ovaries contain an abnormal number of fluid-filled follicles.

Having two of the three criteria may mean you have PCOS.

Despite the name of the disorder, women with PCOS do not actually produce cysts, but rather refer to follicles that are unable to release an egg. This is a sign that ovulation does not happen. PCOS may be caused due to abnormal hormone levels within the body, thus disrupting reproductive functions.

The main reason why ovarian cysts are confused with PCOS is because they share symptoms, namely the abnormal changes to periods, pelvic pain and nausea. They also refer to cysts being the central issue that causes complications. However, PCOS is actually a disruption of hormonal balance that causes significant changes to a woman's reproductive functions. Ovarian cysts, on the other hand, form as a result of the menstrual cycle, and do not disrupt reproductive functions. Ovarian cysts can cause major physical complications such as ovarian torsion, while PCOS causes physical changes due to the ongoing hormonal imbalance.

In some cases, those with PCOS may not develop any ovarian cysts at all.

Section 7

Management/Treatment of Ovarian Cysts

Approach Considerations

Many patients with simple ovarian cysts based on ultrasonographic findings do not require treatment. In a postmenopausal patient, a persistent simple cyst smaller than 10cm in dimension in the presence of a normal CA125 value may be monitored with serial ultrasonographic examinations.

Premenopausal women with asymptomatic simple cysts smaller than 8cm on sonograms in whom the CA125 value is within the reference range may be monitored, with a repeat ultrasonographic examination in 8-12 weeks. Hormone therapy, including, as stated above, the use of the OCPs, is not helpful in resolving the cyst.

Many patients with simple ovarian cysts found through ultrasonographic examination do not require treatment. In a postmenopausal patient, a persistent simple cyst smaller than 10 cm in dimension in the presence of a normal CA125 value may be monitored with serial ultrasonographic examinations.

Ovarian Cysts Can Resolve naturally

Sometimes. Some small ovarian cysts, such as functional cysts, may resolve on their own without any treatment. However, Not all ovarian cysts heal naturally, as the treatment of ovarian cysts depends on several factors, including the size, type, and symptoms of the cyst. Larger cysts or cysts that are causing significant pain or discomfort may require medical intervention.

Additionally, some ovarian cysts, such as dermoid cysts or endometriomas, will not go away on their own and may require surgery to remove. Remember, it is important to consult your doctor if you have an ovarian cyst, as they can provide an accurate diagnosis and recommend appropriate treatment options based on your individual situation.

Home remedies for an ovarian cyst

Women who suspect ovarian cysts should see a doctor before trying any home treatments, as it is essential to diagnose the cause of the cyst and then curate the treatment plan accordingly.

Some natural remedies may help alleviate symptoms of ovarian cysts, but it's important to consult with a doctor before trying any new treatments.

1. **Over-the-counter analgesics:** Some over-the-counter pain medications can temporarily relieve pain. However, you must consult your doctor if the pain persists or comes back too often.

2. **Heat therapy:** Applying a heating pad or warm compress to the lower abdomen may help alleviate pelvic pain and cramping caused by ovarian cysts.

3. **Epsom salt bath:** Taking an Epsom salt bath can help women reduce the pain and other symptoms of ovarian cysts. The high concentration of magnesium sulphate in Epsom salt acts as a muscle relaxant, relieving pain.

4. **Relaxation techniques:** Some relaxation techniques, such as deep breathing, meditation, yoga, etc., can help manage the symptoms of ovarian cysts, as stress and anxiety can exacerbate symptoms such as pain and discomfort.

5. **Exercise:** Regular exercise can help improve blood flow and reduce inflammation, which may help reduce the risk of ovarian cysts and improve overall ovarian health.

6. **Dietary changes:** Eating a balanced diet with plenty of fruits, vegetables, whole grains, and lean protein may help support overall reproductive health.

7. **Herbal remedies:** Some herbs, such as ginger and turmeric, may have anti-inflammatory properties that could help reduce inflammation and pain associated with ovarian cysts. Curcumin or turmeric has been shown to help with PCOS and ovarian cysts. According to a scientific study, ginger exhibits phytotherapeutic and medicinal characteristics. These mostly include antimicrobial, anti-inflammatory, and

antioxidant properties. As a result, the versatile herb helps to diminish hormonal dominance in various ways. It's important to consult your doctor before taking any herbal supplements, as they may interact with other medications or have side effects.

Remember, while these remedies may help alleviate symptoms associated with ovarian cysts, they are not a substitute for medical treatment. It's important to consult your doctor to determine the best course of treatment for your individual situation.

Pharmacologic therapy

Oral contraceptive pills (OCPs) protect against the development of functional ovarian cysts. Existing functional cysts, however, do not regress more quickly when treated with combined oral contraceptives than they do with expectant management.

Laparotomy and laparoscopy

Persistent simple ovarian cysts larger than 10 cm (especially if symptomatic) and complex ovarian cysts should be considered for surgical removal. The surgical approaches include an open technique (laparotomy) or a minimally invasive technique (laparoscopy) with very small incisions. The latter approach is preferred in cases presumed benign. Removing the cyst intact for pathologic analysis may mean removing the entire ovary, though a fertility sparing surgery should be attempted in younger women.

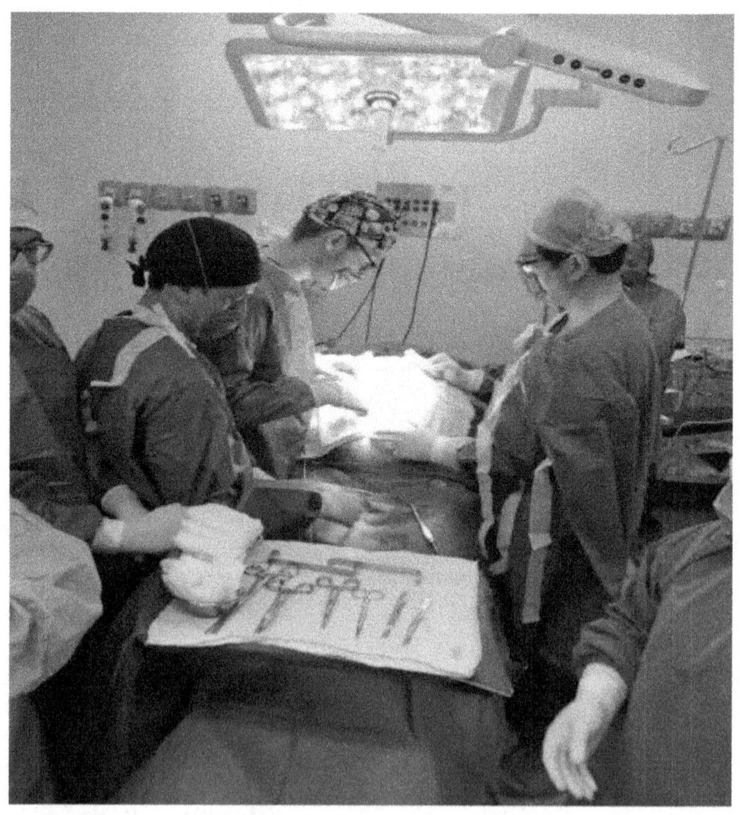

Bilateral oophorectomy

Bilateral oophorectomy and, often, hysterectomy are performed in many postmenopausal women with ovarian cysts, because of the increased incidence of neoplasms in this population.

Referral

Per ACOG Guidelines, referral to a gynecologic oncologist is recommended for the following patients:

- Postmenopausal patient with elevated CA125, imaging findings consistent with malignancy, ascites, a nodular or fixed mass, or evidence of metastases
- Premenopausal patient with very elevated CA125, imaging findings consistent with malignancy, ascites, a nodular or fixed mass, or evidence of metastases
- Premenopausal or postmenopausal patient with elevated malignancy predictive score such as the multivariate index assay, risk of malignancy index, or the Risk of Ovarian Malignancy Algorithm, or one of the ultrasound-based scoring systems from the International Ovarian Tumor Analysis Group.

Section 8

Prevention of Ovarian Cysts

There is no effective means of preventing ovarian cysts from occurring. After an ovarian cyst has disappeared, with or without medical treatment, follow up checks will be done to make sure there is no recurrence. Regular checks can be very important in catching potential recurrence early, which can help in quickly remediating the matter and with little to no surgery required (if it is not malignant). Some doctors do recommend low dose hormonal contraceptives as a way to prevent a recurrence, despite there being little to no evidence of its actual efficacy.

Be sure to notify the doctor if you or your loved one experiences any changes, such as changes to the menstrual cycle, the presence of any pelvic pain or discomfort, or the recurrence of any other symptoms of an ovarian cyst. Lifestyle changes may or may not help in preventing recurrences; this includes quitting smoking, having healthier meals, and regular exercise.

Section 9

FAQ on Ovarian Cysts

Does an ovarian cyst cause pain?

The majority of individuals with ovarian cysts are asymptomatic, and the cysts are frequently detected by chance during routine pelvic exams or ultrasonography. Nevertheless, some cysts may cause a variety of symptoms, which can sometimes be severe. Malignant ovarian cysts, on the other hand, often do not present symptoms until they have progressed to an advanced stage. In this article, we will learn if ovarian cysts always cause pain and how they cause pain.

How can an ovarian cyst cause pain?

Ovarian cysts can lead to pain in a few ways. The pain associated with ovarian cysts is often mostly due to the pressure of the tissues surrounding the ovary. Depending on the size and location of the cyst, it can put pressure on the surrounding organs and nerves. In some cases, ovarian cysts can trigger dull and aching lower back pain.

Additionally, if an ovarian cyst bursts or ruptures or gets twisted, it can cause pain. A ruptured cyst can cause sudden, sharp pain in the lower abdomen or back, abdominal bloating, and vaginal spotting or bleeding, among other symptoms. Moreover, it can also cause pain during sex or dyspareunia.

The most common drugs given to relieve pain with an ovarian cyst are nonsteroidal anti-inflammatory drugs (NSAIDs). These are over-the-counter pain relievers, such as ibuprofen or naproxen, that can help relieve pain caused by ovarian cysts.

Remember, if you experience persistent or severe pelvic pain, it's essential to speak with your doctor to determine the underlying cause and appropriate treatment.

How much weight can an ovarian cyst have?

Ovarian cysts vary in weight, and the weight and size of ovarian cysts are linked. Small ovarian cysts are usually asymptomatic and discovered incidentally through clinical examination or ultrasound. They may occasionally cause pain or discomfort. Certain ovarian cysts can grow abnormally large in rare cases. The contents of a cyst are the most important factors in determining its weight. The cellular components and fluid content make up the cystic composition. While the size of the cystic mass can be determined by the imaging scans of the ovarian cyst. Older women have a chance of developing these giant ovarian cysts. There have also been reports of large ovarian cysts weighing 148.6 and 79.4 kg.

What symptoms are associated with giant ovarian cysts?

Ovarian cysts can grow quite large in rare cases. These are known as giant ovarian cystic masses. Patients with small cysts are frequently asymptomatic until the tumor becomes large enough to have a mass effect on the surrounding organs. The cyst can originate from a variety of locations, making it difficult to pinpoint its source prior to surgery. A giant ovarian cyst's mass effect can cause a variety of non-specific symptoms such as abdominal bloating, nausea, and constipation. Giant ovarian cysts are extremely rare; however, when they do occur, surgical removal is required due to not only the morbidity and mortality associated with the mass effect but also the risk of malignancy.

What are the risks of having abnormally giant ovarian cysts?

Giant abdominal cystic masses are uncommon and necessitate surgical excision due to the symptoms they cause. However, the complications associated with such large cysts are numerous, including bowel obstruction, vomiting, pain, nausea, and distension.

The most serious complication is rupturing, which can result in severe upper pelvic or lower abdominal pain. Another complication associated with ovarian cysts is ovarian torsion, which causes upper pelvic or lower abdominal pain. Another complication associated with ovarian cysts is ovarian torsion. Ovarian torsion occurs when a cyst grows large enough to cause the ovary to twist on its own blood vessels, occasionally halting blood flow. This complication necessitates immediate surgery. If not treated promptly, the twisted ovary can die, causing the person to become very ill and lose the ovary. Please remember that complications such as ovarian rupture and torsion will be excruciatingly painful and necessitate medical attention.

Why did my ovarian cyst grow back?

Most ovarian cysts are functional, but complex ovarian cysts have the potential to grow and lead to severe complications. Despite the fact that the precise cause of these abnormal cystic growths is unknown, a number of risk factors, such as hormonal imbalances, severe pelvic infections, pregnancy, endometriosis, and even PCOS, have been connected to them.

Ovarian cysts are a common occurrence in women. Functional ovarian cysts are a common occurrence during the menstrual cycle. These cysts typically have no symptoms and disappear in a matter of weeks.

Dermoid cysts, cystadenomas, and endometriomas are a few less frequent types of cysts. These cysts may develop further and cause serious complications. Cystic growth is one of them, and it might be a key sign of the underlying malignancy. Although the exact cause of these abnormal cystic growths is unknown, a number of risk factors have been linked to them, including hormonal imbalances, severe pelvic infections, pregnancy, endometriosis, and even PCOS. As a result, this article provides a summary of the various warning signs, diagnostic clues, and preventative measures for developing ovarian cysts.

What warning signs point to the growth of the ovarian cyst?

Simple or functional ovarian cysts typically have no symptoms. However, dermoids and cystadenomas are examples of complex ovarian cysts that can enlarge uncontrollably. This might move your ovary out of position. Besides that, it may result in ovarian torsion, a painful condition where your ovary has twisted. When a cyst bursts, it may result in vomiting, bleeding, rapid breathing, weakness, fever, dizziness, and severe abdominal pain. Additionally, cysts can squeeze your bladder, resulting in frequent or urgent urination.

How can the growth of ovarian cysts be assessed?

An ultrasound scan may reveal a cyst, in which case a gynecologist will likely need to monitor it and conduct another scan a few weeks later. In addition, if there is any suspicion that the cystic mass may be cancerous, the doctor will advise confirmation blood tests to check for specific substances that can indicate ovarian cancer.

The presence of these chemicals in high concentrations, however, is not always a sign of cancer because they can also be brought on by non-cancerous conditions like endometriosis, a pelvic infection, fibroids, or even your period.

How can the growth of ovarian cysts be prevented?

Ovarian cyst development cannot be stopped, especially in women of childbearing age. However, early ovarian cyst detection is possible with routine gynecological exams. Usually, ovarian cysts that aren't cancerous don't develop into cancer. Even so, ovarian cancer symptoms can resemble those of an ovarian cyst. Therefore, it's crucial to see a doctor and get a proper diagnosis. It may be beneficial to maintain a healthy weight, lead a healthy lifestyle, and be aware of the warning signs. Always talk to your doctor if your menstrual cycle changes, you have persistent pelvic pain, you lose your appetite, you lose weight suddenly, or you feel full in your stomach.

Can ovarian cysts be treated without surgery?

Yes, most functional and noncancerous ovarian cysts are asymptomatic. They typically disappear on their own. However, those that don't, need to be closely monitored. The cyst may require surgical removal if it becomes large, painful, or appears to be cancerous. However, these ovarian cysts cannot be treated by some at-home remedies, which may only help with prevention and symptom relief.

Formations on the ovaries that contain liquid are called ovarian cysts. These come in both cancerous and non-cancerous forms. However, it's possible that you are unaware that you have ovarian cysts. This is because many don't show any symptoms and may go away by themselves. Nevertheless, one should see a doctor if they have severe pelvic or abdominal pain, along with a fever and vomiting. Considering the significance of the condition, this article discusses nonsurgical treatment options as well as at-home measures that may help ease the symptoms.

How are ovarian cysts non-surgically treated?

The course of treatment for an ovarian cyst typically depends on the cyst's size and nature, appearance, accompanying symptoms, and the patient's age. The cysts are typically not cancerous and frequently go away within a few months. A subsequent ultrasound scan could be used to confirm that it has resolved. The term "watchful waiting," also known as the "wait-and-see approach," refers to the routine observation of functional ovarian cysts by a physician.

Due to a marginally increased risk of ovarian cancer, women who have undergone menopause may be advised to undergo ultrasound scans and blood tests every four months for a year. The majority of the time, additional tests and treatment are not required if the scans reveal that the cyst has disappeared. If the cyst persists and begins to show signs of cancer, surgery might be advised.

Can you feel by hand if you have a cyst in your ovaries?

No, not always. Ovarian functional cysts typically don't cause any symptoms and disappear on their own. However, sometimes these cysts do not go away, and in these instances, there is pelvic or abdominal pain. The ovarian cyst typically turns into a medical emergency when the pain is accompanied by nausea, a fever, and other symptoms resembling shock.

The cystic developments on or around the ovaries are generally not noticeable. And these tiny, tissue- or fluid-filled pouches on or inside your ovaries are actually quite typical. However, an ovarian cyst might be the cause of persistent, severe abdominal pain or other symptoms that don't seem quite normal. Hence, this article lists the typical symptoms of ovarian cysts as well as those that require medical attention and the risk factors related to them because ignoring them could result in serious health problems.

When should someone with ovarian cysts seek medical attention?

You should seek assistance right away if you experience severe pelvic pain, particularly if it comes on suddenly. The sooner you seek medical attention, the better chance there is for your ovary to be saved because a twisted ovary can reduce or stop blood flow. Furthermore, one should seek emergency medical attention if the abdominal pain is accompanied by a fever, vomiting, cold, clammy skin, rapid breathing, lightheadedness, or weakness.

Does the ovarian cyst have a physical sensation outside the body?

No, not always. Ovarian cysts are frequently found during a standard examination involving both a clinical examination and ultrasonography. Transvaginal ultrasonography is the preferred method of detection; however, a clinical examination that includes a pelvic exam may not be very effective. Cysts should be routinely monitored as they have a chance of turning cancerous.

Ovarian cysts, which are liquid sacs, can form in or on your ovaries. Most noncancerous or cancerous ovarian cysts are brought on by hormonal changes, pregnancy, or diseases like endometriosis. Please remember that the most common type of ovarian cyst, an ovulatory or functional cyst, is entirely normal. It expands each month when you ovulate. They usually don't cause any harm, don't show any symptoms, and go away on their own in a few weeks. These ovarian cysts do, however, have the capacity to grow and cause serious complications. This article gives a general overview of the significance of cyst size, how cysts are evaluated, and how cyst size influences how they are treated.

Is it possible to feel an ovarian cyst outside the body?

No, not always. Ovarian cysts are typically fluid-filled lumps that can develop on one or both ovaries at any time during a woman's lifetime. Sometimes they are solid; in that case, they are referred to as tumors, which is a medical term for "swelling."

Ovarian cysts are frequently discovered by doctors during a routine examination. Pelvic examination is typically part of the clinical checkup. Clinical examination, however, might not be very helpful in detecting them; transvaginal ultrasonography is the imaging method of choice. Once identified cysts need to be treated as soon as possible because they have the potential to be cancerous. The majority of cysts, however, are not cancerous.

Which ovarian cyst sizes and types are there?

Ovarian cysts come in a variety of forms, each with its own causes and characteristics. Depending on the type of cyst, an ovarian cyst's size can also keep changing.

When your menstrual cycle adheres to the prescribed schedule, functional cysts develop. However, the cyst might occasionally keep growing. These primarily consist of corpus luteum and follicular cysts. The majority of functional cysts are between 2 and 5 centimeters, Ovulation takes place when these cysts are 2 to 3 cm in size. Some, however, might grow to be 8 to 12 cm in size.

Those that are abnormally large are pathological ovarian cysts. These primarily consist of dermoid cysts, a type of ovarian tumor that typically progresses at a rate of 1.8 mm and infrequently reaches a size of 15 cm. Cystadenomas can also grow to be quite large. Some can reach a height of 30 cm and range in size from 1 to 3 cm. Finally, although endometriomas are typically small, they can range in size like other cysts.

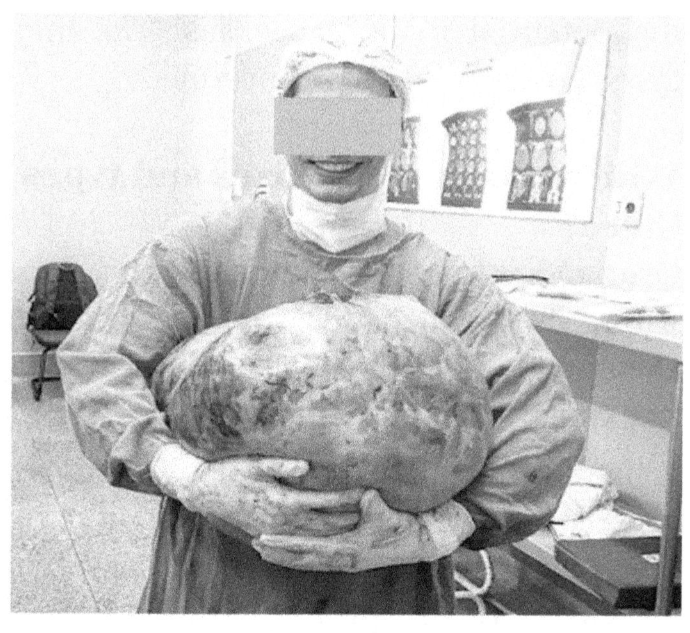

How are ovarian cysts handled medically?

Many ovarian cysts resolve on their own and don't need to be treated. As a result, your doctor might advise a period of "watchful waiting," during which you should keep an eye on your cyst to see if it disappears after one or two menstrual cycles.

Your doctor might advise prescribing pain relievers if you experience discomfort due to an ovarian cyst. In addition, a cyst's size may determine whether it needs to be surgically removed.

Surgery is typically not advised for noncancerous ovarian cysts unless they measure more than 10 centimeters. However, this rule is not set in stone. For instance, a simple cyst might not require treatment until it measures 10 cm or 4 inches. Besides that, when cancerous cysts are much smaller, they may be removed.

Ovarian cysts are frequently surgically removed using minimally invasive techniques like laparoscopy. However, when a cyst is very large or cancer is suspected, more extensive open surgery may be required. A prescribed hormonal contraceptive may be recommended to you by your doctor if you frequently develop functional cysts. This medication won't shrink an existing cyst, but it can aid in preventing the development of brand-new functional cysts.